The Vibrant Ketogenic Diet Snack & Desserts Recipes

Quick and Easy Irresistible Recipes Affordable for Beginners and Busy People

Michelle Lewis

© Copyright 2021 - All rights reserved.

The content contained within this book may not be reproduced, duplicated or transmitted without direct written permission from the author or the publisher.

Under no circumstances will any blame or legal responsibility be held against the publisher, or author, for any damages, reparation, or monetary loss due to the information contained within this book. Either directly or indirectly.

Legal Notice:

This book is copyright protected. This book is only for personal use. You cannot amend, distribute, sell, use, quote or paraphrase any part, or the content within this book, without the consent of the author or publisher.

Disclaimer Notice:

Please note the information contained within this document is for educational and entertainment purposes only. All effort has been executed to present accurate, up to date, and reliable, complete information. No warranties of any kind are declared or implied. Readers acknowledge that the author is not engaging in the rendering of legal, financial, medical or professional advice. The content within this book has been derived from various sources. Please consult a licensed professional before attempting any techniques outlined in this book.

By reading this document, the reader agrees that under no circumstances is the author responsible for any losses, direct or indirect, which are incurred as a result of the use of information contained within this document, including, but not limited to, — errors, omissions, or inaccuracies.

Contents

Chocolate Japanese Cheesecake

Preparation Time: 20 minutes

Cooking Time: 40 minutes

Servings: 8

Ingredients:

- 3 pieces egg
- 120 g Cream Cheese (Philadelphia)
- 100g Sugar Free Chocolate
- ½ tsp Lemon juice

Directions:

1. Preheat your oven to 170 ° C (top and bottom heat, without convection) and place a pan with water on the bottom. Cover the bottom and sides of the 20 cm baking dish with parchment and grease it with oil; Wrap foil outside.
2. Separate the whites from the yolks. Beat the proteins at low speed until foam; add lemon juice and beat at high speed until steady peaks.
3. Melt your chocolate in water bath, add cream cheese to it and mix until smooth. Remove from heat, cool slightly, add yolks and mix thoroughly.

4. Gently add the proteins to the chocolate mixture (one-third at a time), mix and pour the dough into a baking dish.

5. Place the pan directly on a baking sheet with water and cook for 15 minutes. Then lower the temperature to 150 ° C and cook for another 20 minutes. Turn off the oven and leave the cheesecake in it for another 20 minutes.

Nutrition:

135 Calories

11g Fat

6g Carbohydrate

4g Fiber

4g Protein

Italian Cream Cake

Preparation Time: 30 minutes

Cooking Time: 1 hour

Servings: 4

Ingredients:

For the Cake

- Two cups of almond flour
- One cup of coconut flour
- One cup of softened butter that is unsalted
- 4 very big eggs
- 1 cup of erythritol
- A pinch of salt
- 2 table spoon of baking powder
- One cup of heavy cream
- Half table spoon of cream of tartar
- One table spoon of vanilla extract
- One cup of pecans (already chopped)
- One cup of already shredded coconut

For the frosting

- Half cup of heavy cream
- One cup of soft butter that is unsalted
- Two table spoons of vanilla extract
- One cup of cream cheese
- Half cup of swerve (powdered)

- For the garnish
- Two table spoons of pecans that are chopped already
- Two table spoons of shredded coconut that are toasted

Directions:

1. Before starting the preparation, first heat the oven to about 350F. Use the parchment paper lining to line the inside of the cake baking pan and grease it with a little butter for easy remover
2. Add the flour, the baking powder, the salt and the pecans and coconut into a large bowl and stir. In another bowl, put the sweetener and the butter and cream it until it becomes very fluffy and light.
3. Remove the yolks from the egg and beat them. Then add to the mixture of sweetener and butter and mix it well. Then add the heavy cream and the vanilla to the above mixture and mix it very well again.
4. Add the dry ingredients (the almond flour, the coconut flour, the salt and the baking powder) in to the mixed butter mixture and stir until it

is fully combined. Put the egg whites of the already removed yolk into a bowl and whisk it together with the cream of tartar. Mix it well until it foams.

5. Then fold this mixture into the already mixed barter. To make the batter light, be sure to fold the egg white mixture lightly.

6. Pour the battered mixture into the baking pan and allow it to bake for about 40 minutes in the already heated oven. By this time, the edges of the cake should be a shade of golden brown and the center of the cake should be firm.

7. Leave it in the baking pans to cool. Remove the cake from the pans when they are already cool.

8. For the frosting

9. Put the cream cheese and the butter together in a mixing bowl and start to mix them until the mixture becomes very fluffy and light.

10. To the mixture, add the sweetener and the vanilla and mix it by beating the mixture.

11. Next, add the heavy cream to the mixture. To get your desired consistency, add the heavy cream slowly so as to be able to stop when it reaches the desired consistency.

12. Paste the top of the cake and the side of the cake with the frosting.

13. On the top layer of the cake, sprinkle the roasted coconut that was shredded and use to decorate the cake.

Nutrition:

40g Carbohydrates

0g Dietary Fiber

28g Sugar

30g Fat

Fudge Ice Pops

Preparation Time: 80 minutes

Cooking Time: 0 minute

Servings: 4

Ingredients

- ½ (13.5-ounce) can coconut cream
- 2 teaspoons Swerve natural sweetener
- 2 tablespoons unsweetened cocoa powder
- 2 tablespoons sugar-free chocolate chips

Directions:

1. In a food processor (or blender), mix together the coconut cream, sweetener, and unsweetened cocoa powder. Pour into ice pop molds and drop chocolate chips into each mold. Freeze for at least 2 hours before serving.

Nutrition:

193 Calories

9g Carbs

2g Protein

Orange Cream Float

Preparation Time: 90 minutes

Cooking Time: 0 minute

Serves: 2

Ingredients

- 1 can Stevia orange soda
- 4 tablespoons heavy (whipping) cream
- 1 teaspoon vanilla extract
- 6 ice cubes

Directions:

1. Combine all the ingredients: in your blender and process until combines and frothy. Blend well, pour into two tall glasses, and serve.

Nutrition:

56 Calories

3g Carbs

1g Protein

Root Beer Float

Preparation Time: 5 minutes

Cooking Time: 0 minute

Servings: 2

Ingredients

- 1 (12-ounce) can diet root beer
- 4 tablespoons heavy (whipping) cream
- 1 teaspoon vanilla extract
- 6 ice cubes

Directions:

1. Combine all the ingredients: in your blender and process until smooth. Pour into two tall glasses and serve.

Nutrition:

56 Calories

3g Carbs

1g Protein

Chocolate Fat Bombs

Preparation Time: 10 minutes

Cooking Time: 5 minutes

Servings: 15

Ingredients:

- 1/2 cup coconut butter, softened
- 1/4 cup extra virgin coconut oil, softened
- 1/2 cup butter, softened
- 3 tablespoons unsweetened cacao powder
- 15 to 20 drops liquid stevia
- Optional: 2 tablespoons Erythritol or Swerve, powdered
- Optional: 1 teaspoon hazelnut, cherry, or almond extract, or pinch of cayenne pepper

Directions:

1. Incorporate all ingredients in a food processor, reserving some cacao aside for coating. Process until smooth. Line a baking sheet with parchment paper.
2. With a spoon, make 15 small truffles. Chill for 60 minutes.
3. Remove the baking sheet from the fridge. Mix in remaining cacao powder over the fat bombs.

4. Prep Air Fryer to 350 degrees F to preheat. Situate Air Fryer basket with space in between each and set to air fry for 5 minutes.

Nutrition:

143 Calories

2.7g Carbs

0.9g Protein

Coffee Fat Bombs

Preparation Time: 10 minutes

Cooking Time: 5 minutes

Servings: 6

Ingredients:

- 1/4 cup extra virgin coconut oil, softened
- 1/2 cup butter or more coconut oil, softened
- 3 tablespoons unsweetened coffee powder
- 15 to 20 drops liquid stevia
- Optional: 2 tablespoons Erythritol or Swerve, powdered
- 1 teaspoon hazelnut or almond extract, or pinch of cayenne pepper
- 1/2 cup coconut butter, softened

Direction:

1. Mix all the ingredients in a food processor, reserving some coffee aside for coating. Blend until smooth. Prep baking sheet with a parchment paper.
2. With a spoon, make 15 small truffles. Chill for 40 minutes.
3. Remove the fat bombs from the fridge and sprinkle with remaining coffee powder.

4. Ready Air Fryer to preheat to 350 degrees F. Arrange the truffles into your Air Fryer basket, leaving space between each.

5. Set to air fry for 5 minutes.

Nutrition:

110 calories

10g fats

21g protein

Berry Cheesecake Fat Bombs

Preparation Time: 90 minutes

Cooking Time: 0 minute

Servings: 2

Ingredients:

- 4 ounces cream cheese, softened
- 4 tablespoons butter, softened
- 2 teaspoons Swerve natural sweetener
- 1 teaspoon vanilla extract
- ¼ cup berries, fresh or frozen

Directions:

1. In a medium bowl, use a hand mixer to beat the cream cheese, butter, sweetener, and vanilla. In a small bowl, mash the berries thoroughly.
2. Fold the berries into the cream-cheese mixture using a rubber scraper.
3. Spoon the cream-cheese mixture into fat bomb molds.
4. Freeze for at least 2 hours, unmold them, and eat! Leftover fat bombs can be stored in the freezer in a zip-top bag for up to 3 months.

Nutrition:

414 Calories

9g Carbs

4g Protein

Sweet Fat Bombs

Preparation Time: 25 minutes

Cooking Time: 7 minutes

Servings: 12

Ingredients:

- 5 tablespoon swerves
- 6 tablespoon peanut butter, melted
- ½ teaspoon vanilla extract
- ¼ teaspoon salt
- 6 tablespoon Erythritol
- 1 teaspoon stevia extract
- 8 tablespoon fresh lemon juice
- 3 eggs
- 1 teaspoon lime zest
- 2 tablespoon coconut oil

Directions:

1. Mix together the peanut butter and swerve. Add the vanilla extract, Erythritol and salt and beat well.
2. Place the peanut butter mixture in truffle forms. Place the peanut mixture in freezer.

3. Preheat the air fryer to 350 F. Mix together the stevia, lemon juice, lime zest, and coconut oil in the bowl.

4. After this, pour the lemon mixture in the air fryer basket and cook it for 5 minutes. Stir it every 2 minutes.

5. Now, crack the eggs in the lemon mixture and mix it with a hand mixer until smooth. Now, set the air fryer to 365 F and cook for 2 minutes more.

6. Remove the curd mixture from air fryer and refrigerate to chill. In a pastry bag, place the curd mixture. Remove truffle from the freezer. Fill each truffle with curd mixture. Place the bomb in a cold place. Enjoy!

Nutrition:

231 Calories

10.3g Carbs

3.5g Protein

Peanut Butter Fat Bombs

Preparation Time: 40 minutes

Cooking Time: 0 minute

Servings: 2

Ingredients:

- 1 tablespoon butter, at room temperature
- 1 tablespoon coconut oil
- 2 tablespoons all-natural peanut butter
- 2 teaspoons Swerve natural sweetener

Directions:

1. In a microwave-safe medium bowl, melt the butter, coconut oil, and peanut butter in the microwave on 50 percent power.
2. Mix in the sweetener. Pour the mixture into fat bomb molds.
3. Freeze for 30 minutes, unmold them, and eat! Keep some extras in your freezer so you can eat them anytime you are craving a sweet treat.

Nutrition:

196 Calories

8g Carbs

3g Protein

Lemonade Fat Bombs

Preparation Time: 90 minutes

Cooking Time: 0 minute

Servings: 4

Ingredients

- ½ lemon
- 4 ounces cream cheese, at room temperature
- 2 ounces butter, at room temperature
- 2 teaspoons Swerve natural sweetener
- Pinch pink salt

Directions:

1. Zest the lemon half with a very fine grater into a small bowl. Squeeze the juice from the lemon half into the bowl with the zest.
2. In a medium bowl, combine the cream cheese and butter. Add the sweetener, lemon zest and juice, and pink salt.
3. Using a hand mixer, beat until fully combined. Spoon the mixture into the fat bomb molds.
4. Freeze for at least 2 hours, unmold, and eat!
5. Keep extras in your freezer in a zip-top bag so you and your loved ones can have them anytime you are craving a sweet treat. They will keep in the freezer for up to 3 months.

Nutrition:

404 Calories

8g Carbs

4g Protein

Creamy Choco Mousse

Preparation Time: 5 minutes

Cooking Time: 0 minute

Servings: 4

Ingredients:

- 1 cup of creamed coconut milk
- ½ tsp. of cinnamon
- Shredded coconut for garnish
- 3 tbsp. of raw cocoa powder
- 6-12 drops of liquid stevia extract

Directions:

1. Put a coconut milk can into your fridge overnight.
2. Once thick, put it into a bowl. Whip in raw cocoa powder.
3. Add in cinnamon and stevia. Whip until it's smooth and creamy.
4. Place in serving glass then garnish using some pinch of shredded coconut. Enjoy!

Nutrition:

218 Calories

13.5g Carbohydrates

6.2g Protein

Ginger Bread Cake Roll

Preparation Time: 30 minutes

Cooking Time: 1 hour

Servings: 4

Ingredients:

For the cake

- Half cup of almond flour
- One table spoon of ethical approval
- A quarter cup of a powdered sweetener
- Half tablespoon of grass-fed gelatin
- One eighth table spoon of cream of tarter
- A quarter table spoon of powdered ginger
- A pinch of salt
- A little cinnamon powder
- A quarter table spoon of vanilla extract
- One eight of powdered cloves
- One large egg

For the vanilla cream filling

- One cup of softened cream cheese
- Half cup of whipping cream
- Two table spoon of powdered sweetener
- A quarter tablespoon of vanilla extract

Directions:

1. For the cake

2. Heat the oven to 350F before starting the cake preparation process. Place a parchment paper in a baking pan and line the baking pan with it. Use a little butter to grease the sides of the baking pan and also the parchment paper.

3. Whisk the almond flour, the cocoa powder, the powdered sweetener, ginger, gelatin, powdered cloves together in a medium mixing bowl.

4. Get another mixing bowl and mix the granulated sugar together with the egg yolk until the mixture gets thickened and the color turns light yellow.

5. Also add the vanilla extract and beat the mixture well.

6. Beat the egg whites and the cream of tartar and a little salt together in another mixing bowl until the mixture becomes frothy. When it is already frothy, add the remaining sweetener and beat it well.

7. Fold the beat egg yolks into the beat egg whites gently. Then fold this into the almond flour mixture. Be careful not to make it deflated.

8. Make the batter spread in to the already greased baking pan and bake for 12 minutes, until it springs back when the top is touched.

9. Take it away from the oven and let it get cooled a little before removing it. You can to remove it by using a knife to make the edges loosen. Cover the cake with another piece of parchment paper and also use a kitchen towel to cover it. Put another baking sheet that is large on top of it and flip the cake over.

10. Peel the parchment paper gently from the cake and also roll up the kitchen towel gently and let the cake cool down.

11. For the vanilla cream filling

12. Beat half of the whipping cream with the cream cheese in a mixing bowl. Beat it till it becomes smooth.

13. Beat the remaining whipping cream and the sweetener in a big mixing bowl. Then add the vanilla extract and the mixture of the whipping cream and beat very well, but do not over beat it. Keep about half of the mixture to decorate the cake.

14. Unroll the cake carefully. Let the cake curl up on the ends and do not lay it down flat completely.

15. Spread the rest of the filling on the cake and roll it up back gently. Do not roll it up back with the kitchen towel.

16. Place it on a serving plate. Place the seam side down. Put the remaining cream mixture on the center of the cake in different shapes. You can use an icing pipe to achieve desired shapes.

17. Keep In the refrigerator.

Nutrition:

206 calories

18.06g Fat

5.68g Protein

3.99g Carbohydrate

Ketogenic Pumpkin Cheese Cake

Preparation Time: 30 minutes

Cooking Time: 1 hour

Servings: 4

Ingredients:

For the crust

- A quarter cup of almond flour
- Half table spoon of melted butter
- One table spoon of powdered sweetener
- A pinch of salt
- A quarter table spoon of powdered ginger
- A quarter table spoon of cinnamon powder

For the pumpkin cheese cake

- A cup of softened cheese
- One egg
- Half a cup of softened cream cheese
- Half table spoon of pumpkin pie spice
- Three table spoons of pumpkin puree
- Half tablespoon of vanilla extract

Directions:

1. For the crust
2. Whisk the almond flour, the spices, salt and the sweetener together in a big mixing bowl. Add

the butter that is now melted and stir until the mixture becomes clumpy.

3. Pour the mixture into a spring form baking pan.

4. For the filing

5. Beat the softened cheese and the cream cheese together until it combines well. Add the sweetener and stir well until it becomes smooth.

6. Add the pumpkin pie spice, pumpkin puree, the vanilla extract and combine it well by beating it well. Add the egg and continue beating it until it combines well.

7. Use a large foil paper to wrap the bottom of the spring form pan. Wrap it tightly. Put a paper towel over the pan. Be careful not to make it touch the cake. Then wrap another foil over the cake top. The reason for wrapping with foil is to prevent excess moisture from entering the cake.

8. Bake the cake for about 30 minutes; bring it to cool it down.

9. Refrigerate for about four hours. When it is chilled, use a knife to remove the cake.

10. If you like, you can add a topping of caramel
sauce and whipped cream

Nutrition:

246g Calories

23.4g Fat

5.3g Protein

3.23g Carbohydrates

Cannoli Sheet Cake

Preparation Time: 20 minutes

Cooking Time: 40 minutes

Servings: 5

Ingredients:

- For the sheet cake
- Half cup of almond flour
- Half table spoon of vanilla extract
- A quarter cup of sweetener
- A little water
- Two table spoons of coconut flour
- Three table spoons of melted butter
- Two table spoons of protein powder
- One egg
- A pinch of salt
- Half table spoon of baking powder
- For the cannoli cream frosting
- A quarter cup of milk ricotta
- Two tablespoons of chocolate chips (sugar free)
- Two table spoon of softened cheese cream
- A quarter table spoon of vanilla extract
- A quarter cup of powdered sweetener
- A quarter cup of heavy whipping cream

Directions:

1. Heat the oven to about 325F. Grease a small jelly roll pan to avoid the cake sticking to the bottom of the pan.
2. Whisk the almond flour, coconut flour, sweetener, protein powder, baking powder, and the salt in a big mixing bowl. Add the, already melted butter, eggs, water, and the vanilla extract and stir until they have combined very well.
3. The batter is then poured into the already prepared baking pan and spread it so that there is an even distribution of the batter in the baking pan. Bake the bake for about 22 minutes till the color becomes golden brown and becomes firm while touched.
4. Remove the baking pan from the oven and let cool completely.

Nutrition:

235 calories

20g Fat

6.8g Protein

6.2g Carbohydrates

Coconut Flour

Chocolate Cupcake

Preparation Time: 30 minutes

Cooking Time: 45 minutes

Servings: 4

Ingredients:

- Four table spoons of melted butter
- Three table spoon of cocoa butter
- Three table spoons of almond cream that is unsweetened
- Two eggs
- A pinch of salt
- Three table spoons of sweetener
- One table spoon of baking powder
- One table spoon of vanilla essence
- For the butter cream
- Half cup of sweetener
- One table spoon of instant coffee
- Two table spoons of softened cream cheese
- A little hot water
- Half a cup of whipping cream

Directions:

1. Heat the oven to 370 F Use some parchment paper to line the insides of the muffin tin

2. Add the cocoa powder, melted butter, the espresso powder and melted butter together in a big mixing bowl and whisk them together.

3. Add the vanilla essence and eggs to the mixture then add the baking powder, coconut flour, a pinch of salt and the sweetener, and then beat well to combine it together.

Nutrition:

268 Calories

29g Fat

13g Protein

Classic New York
Ketogenic Cheese Cake

Preparation Time: 1 hour

Cooking Time: 5 hours

Servings: 4

Ingredients:

- 4 table spoons of cream cheese that is already softened
- One table spoon of vanilla extract
- One egg
- Two table spoons of soft butter that is not salted
- One table spoon of lemon zest that is grated
- Five table spoons of powdered sweetener
- Three table spoons of sour cream that is at room temperature

Directions:

1. Get the oven pre heated to about 300F. Get a spring form pan and grease it with butter. Grease it well so that the cake would remove well.
2. Put a parchment paper that is already cut to the shape of the spring form pan in the bottom of

the pan. Grease the parchment paper with butter. Wrap the outside of the pan with aluminum foil paper to cover the bottom of the pan and also to cover the outside of the pan more than half way up.

3. Get a mixing bowl and add the cream cheese and butter and beat it till it becomes smooth. Also add the sweetener and beat till the mixture has combined very well. Add the egg into the mixture and beat again.

4. Put the lemon zest, sour cream and also the vanilla extract and beat it until it is very smooth and it has fully combined. Pour the batter into the already greased spring form pan and smoothen the top of the batter.

5. Put the spring form pan in a big roasting pan so that the sides don't touch. Put the roasting pan in the oven. Pour some boiling water carefully into the roasting pan until it reaches half of the sides.

6. Bake for about 90 minutes and let it cool after baking.

7. When it is cool, carefully remove the cake and refrigerate for 4 hours before serving.

Nutrition:

284 calories

24.7g Fat

2.9g Carbohydrate

5.3g Protein

Slice-And-Bake Vanilla Wafers

Preparation Time: 10 minutes

Cooking Time: 15 minutes

Servings: 2

Ingredients:

- 175g (1¾ cups) blanched Almond flour
- ½ cup granulated Erythritol-based Sweetener
- 1 stick (½ cup) unsalted softened Butter
- 2 tbsp. of Coconut flour
- ¼ tsp. of salt
- ½ tsp. of Vanilla extract

Directions:

1. Beat the sweetener and butter using an electric mixer in a large bowl for 2 minutes until it becomes fluffy and light. Then beat in the salt, vanilla extract, coconut flour, and almond until thoroughly mixed.

2. Evenly spread the dough between two sheets of parchment or wax paper and wrap each portion into a size with a diameter of about 1½ inches. Then wrap in paper and refrigerate for 1-2 hours.

3. Heat the oven to 325° F and line a baking sheet using silicone baking mats or parchment paper.

Slice the dough into ¼- inch slices using a sharp knife. Put the sliced dough on the baking sheets and make sure to leave a 1-inch space between wafers.

4. Place in the oven for about 5 minutes. Slightly flatten the cookies using a flat-bottomed glass. Bake for another 8-10 minutes.

Nutrition:

2.2g Protein

9.3g Fat

2.5g Carbohydrate

Amoretti

Preparation Time: 15 minutes

Cooking Time: 22 minutes

Servings: 2

Ingredients:

- ½ cup of granulated Erythritol-based Sweetener
- 165g (2 cups) sliced Almonds
- ¼ cup of powdered of Erythritol-based sweetener
- 4 large egg whites
- Pinch of salt
- ½ tsp almond extract

Directions:

1. Heat the oven to 300° F and use parchment paper to line 2 baking sheets. Grease the parchment slightly.
2. Process the powdered sweetener, granulated sweetener, and sliced almonds in a food processor until it appears like coarse crumbs.
3. Beat the egg whites plus the salt and almond extracts using an electric mixer in a large bowl until they hold soft peaks. Fold in the almond mixture so that it becomes well combined.

4. Drop spoonful of the dough onto the prepared baking sheet and allow for a space of 1 inch between them. Press a sliced almond into the top of each cookie.

5. Bake in the oven for 22 minutes until the sides becomes brown. They will appear jellylike when they are taken out from the oven but will begin to be firms as it cools down.

Nutrition:

8.8g Fat

5.3g Protein

2.3g Fiber

117 Calories

Peanut Butter Cookies for Two

Preparation Time: 5 minutes

Cooking Time: 12 minutes

Servings: 1

Ingredients:

- 1½ tbsp. of creamy salted Peanut Butter
- 1 tbsp. of unsalted softened Butter
- 2 tsp. of lightly beaten egg
- 2 tbsp. of granulated Erythritol-based Sweetener
- ¼ tsp. of Vanilla extract
- 2 tbsp. of defatted Peanut flour
- Pinch of salt
- 2 tsp. of sugarless Chocolate Chips
- 1/8 tsp. of baking powder

Directions:

1. Heat the oven to 325° F and line a baking sheet with a silicone baking mat or parchment paper.
2. Beat in the sweetener, butter, and peanut butter using an electric mixer in a small bowl until it is thoroughly mixed. Then beat in the vanilla extract and the egg.
3. Add the salt, baking powder, and peanut flour and mix until the dough clumps together. Cut

the dough into two and shape each of them into a ball.

4. Position the dough ball into the coated baking sheets and flatten into a circular shape about ½ inch thick. Garnish the dough tops with a tsp. of chocolate chips. Gently press them into the dough to stick.

5. Bake for 10-12 minutes until golden brown.

Nutrition:

13.2g Fat

5.7g Carbohydrates

4.9g protein

163 Calories

Cream Cheese Cookies

Preparation Time: 15 minutes

Cooking Time: 12 minutes

Servings: 6

Ingredients:

- ¼ cup (½ stick) unsalted softened Butter
- ½ cup (4 oz.) of softened Cream Cheese
- 1 large egg at room temp
- ½ of cup granulated Erythritol-based Sweetener
- 150g (1½ cups) of blanched Almond flour
- 1 tsp. of baking Powder
- ½ tsp. of Vanilla extract
- Powdered Erythritol-based sweetener (for dusting)
- ¼ tsp. of salt

Directions:

1. Heat the oven to 350°F and line with a silicone baking mat or parchment paper.
2. Beat the butter and cream cheese using an electric mixer in a large bowl until it appears smooth. Add the sweetener and keep beating. Beat in the vanilla extract and the egg.

3. Whisk in the salt, baking powder, and almond flour in a medium bowl. Add the flour mixture into the cream cheese and until well incorporated.

4. Drop the dough in spoonful onto the coated baking sheet. Flatten the cookies.

5. Bake for 10-12 minutes. Dust with powdered sweetener when cool.

Nutrition:

13.7g Fat

4.1g Protein

1.5g Fiber

154 Calories

Chewy Double Chocolate Cookies

Preparation Time: 15 minutes

Cooking Time: 12 minutes

Servings: 10

Ingredients:

- 3 tbsp. of Cocoa powder
- 2 tbsp. of (88g) plus ¾ cup blanched Almond flour
- ½ tsp. of baking soda
- 1 tbsp. of grass-fed Gelatin
- ½ tsp. of salt
- ½ stick (¼ cup) unsalted softened Butter
- ½ cup of granulated Erythritol-based sweetener
- 1 large egg at room temp
- ¼ cup of unsalted Creamy Almond Butter
- ½ tsp. of Vanilla extract
- 1/3 cup sugarless Chocolate Chips

Directions:

1. Heat the oven to 350° F and line 2 baking sheets with silicone baking mats or parchment paper.
2. Whisk the gelatin, salt, baking soda, cocoa powder, and almond flour together in a medium bowl.

3. Beat the sweetener, almond butter, and butter with an electric mixer in a large bowl until it is thoroughly mixed. Beat the vanilla extract and the egg. The beat in the almond mixture so that the dough sticks together. Add the chocolate chips and stir.

4. Roll the dough into medium-sized cookies and space them an inch apart. Flatten to about ½ inch thick. Bake for about 12 minutes.

Nutrition:

15.1g Fat

6.9g Carbohydrates

5.5g Protein

180 Calories

Mocha Cream Pie

Preparation Time: 15 minutes

Cooking Time: 5 minutes

Servings: 10

Ingredients:

- 1 cup strongly brewed Coffee at room temp
- 1 Easy Chocolate Pie Crust
- 1 cup heavy Whipping Cream
- 1½ tsp. of grass-fed Gelatin
- 1 tsp. of Vanilla extract
- ¼ cup Cocoa powder
- ½ cup powdered Erythritol-based Sweetener

Directions:

1. Grease a 9-inch glass pie pan or ceramic. Press the crust mixture evenly and firmly to the sides of the greased pan or its bottom. Refrigerate until the filling is prepared.
2. Pour the coffee in a small saucepan and add gelatin. Whisk thoroughly and then place over medium heat. Allow to simmer, whisking from time to time to make sure the gelatin dissolves. Allow to cool for 20 minutes.
3. Add the vanilla extract, cocoa powder, sweetener, and the cream into a large bowl.

Use an electric mixer to beat to that it holds stiff peaks.

4. Add gelatin mixture that has been cooled and then beat until it is well incorporated. Pour over the cooled crust and place in the refrigerator for 3 hours until it becomes firm.

Nutrition:

20.2g Fat

4.7g Protein

3.1g Fiber

218 Calories

Coconut Custard Pie

Preparation Time: 10 minutes

Cooking Time: 50 minutes

Servings: 8

Ingredients:

- 1 cup of heavy Whipping Cream
- ¾ cup of powdered Erythritol-based Sweetener
- ½ cup of full-fat Coconut Milk
- 4 large eggs
- ½ stick (¼ cup) of cooled, unsalted, melted butter
- 1¼ cups of unsweetened shredded coconut
- 3 tbsp. of Coconut flour
- ½ tsp. of baking powder
- ½ tsp. of Vanilla extract
- ¼ tsp. of salt

Directions:

1. Heat the oven to 350° F and grease a 9-inch ceramic pie pan or glass.
2. Place the melted butter, eggs, coconut milk, sweetener, and cream in a blender. Blend well.
3. Add the vanilla extract, baking powder, salt, coconut flour, and a cup of shredded coconut. Continue blending.

4. Empty the mixture into the pie pan and sprinkle with the rest of the shredded coconut. Bake for 40-50 minutes and stop when the center is until jiggly but the sides are set.

5. Take out of the oven and allow it to cool for 30 minutes. Place in the refrigerator and allow to stay for 2 hours before cutting it

Nutrition:

29.5g Fat

6.7g Carbohydrates

5.3g Protein

317 Calories

Dairy-Free Fruit Tarts

Preparation Time: 15 minutes

Cooking Time: 15 minutes

Servings: 2

Ingredients:

- 1 cup Coconut Whipped Cream
- ½ Easy Shortbread Crust (dairy-free option)
- Fresh mint Sprigs
- ½ cup mixed fresh Berries

Directions:

1. Grease two 4" pans with detachable bottoms. Pour the shortbread mixture into pans and firmly press into the edges and bottom of each pan. Refrigerate for 15 minutes.
2. Loosen the crust carefully to remove from the pan.
3. Distribute the whipped cream between the tarts and evenly spread to the sides. Refrigerate for 1-2 hours to make it firm.
4. Use the berries and sprig of mint to garnish each of the tarts

Nutrition:

28.9g Fats

8.3g Carbohydrates

5.8g protein

306 Calories

Strawberry Rhubarb Crisp

Preparation Time: 10 minutes

Cooking Time: 30 minutes

Servings: 2

Ingredients:

Topping Ingredients:

- 1 tbsp. of unsweetened shredded Coconut
- 2½ tbsp. of blanched Almond flour
- 1½ tsp. of finely chopped Pecans
- 1 tbsp. of granulated Erythritol-based Sweetener
- Pinch of salt
- 2 tsp. melted unsalted Butter
- ¼ tsp. of ground Cinnamon

Filling Ingredients:

- 1/3 cup of sliced fresh Strawberries
- ½ cup of chopped fresh Rhubarb
- 1/16 tsp. of Xanthan Gum
- 1 tbsp. of granulated Erythritol-based Sweetener

Directions:

1. Preparing the Topping Ingredients:
2. Heat the oven to 300° F and line a baking sheet with parchment paper.

3. Whisk the cinnamon, pecans, salt, sweetener, coconut, and almond flour in a medium bowl. Add the melted butter into the mixture and stir until the resulting mixture appears like coarse crumbs.

4. Place on the coated baking sheet and firmly press down to make it flat. Bake for 15 minutes then allow it to cool.

5. Preparing the Filling and Assembling Ingredients:

6. Heat the oven to 400° F

7. Add all the filling ingredients in a medium bowl and make sure that you thoroughly mix them. Place into an 8-oz ramekin and cover with foil. Place in the oven to bake for 10-15 minutes.

Nutrition:

135 Calories

11.5g Fats

2.6g Protein

Raspberry Fool

Preparation Time: 15 minutes

Cooking Time: 10 minutes

Servings: 4

Ingredients:

- 2-4 tbsp. of powdered and divided Erythritol-based Sweetener
- 1 cup of thawed frozen Raspberries
- Fresh berries, for garnish
- 1 cup of Whipped Cream

Directions:

1. Process 2 tbsp. of sweetener and berries in a food processor or blender until smooth. Fold in the raspberry puree, leaving some streaks.
2. Pour mixture into four dessert cups. Garnish with the berries.

Nutrition:

20.1g Fats

5.2g Carbohydrates

1.7g Protein

1g Fiber

Strawberries with Coconut Whip

Preparation Time: 10 minutes

Cooking Time: 0 minute

Servings: 4

Ingredients:

- 4 cups Strawberries or other favorite berries
- 2 cans Refrigerated coconut cream
- 1 oz. 70% or darker unsweetened chopped dark chocolate

Directions:

1. Remove the solidified cream from the can of milk and set aside for another time, saving the liquid. Pour it into a mixing container and whip with a hand mixer until it forms stiff peaks (approximately five minutes).
2. Slice the berries and portion into four dishes. Serve with a dollop of the cream. Garnish with the chopped chocolate and a few berries. Serve.

Nutrition:

10g Net Carbohydrates

4g Protein

342 Calories

Almond Blackberry
Chia Pudding

Preparation Time: 15 minutes

Cooking Time: 0 minute

Servings: 2

Ingredients:

- ¼ cup Chia seeds
- Drizzle Raw honey
- 2 tbsp Sliced almonds
- 1 ½ cup Vanilla almond milk
- 6 oz. Fresh blackberries

Directions:

1. Rinse and add the berries into a dish. Crush with a fork until creamy. Pour in the raw honey, milk, and chia seeds. Stir well. Refrigerate for several hours or overnight for the most delicious results.
2. Sprinkle with the almonds and several blackberries. Serve any time.

Nutrition:

1g Net Carbohydrates

2g Protein

109 Calories

Choco Mug Brownie

Preparation Time: 10 minutes

Cooking Time: 30 seconds

Servings: 1

Ingredients:

- 1 tbsp Cocoa powder
- ½ tsp Baking powder
- 1 scoop Chocolate protein powder
- ¼ cup Almond milk

Directions:

1. Prepare a mug using the protein powder, cocoa, and baking powder. Pour the milk into the mug and stir. Microwave for about 30 seconds and serve.

Nutrition:

12.4g Protein

15.8g Total Fats

207 Calories

Chocolate Mousse

Preparation Time: 1 hour

Cooking Time: 0 minute

Servings: 2

Ingredients:

- 4 tbsp Butter
- 4 tbsp Cream Cheese
- 1 ½ tbsp Heavy whipping cream
- 1 tbsp Swerve or another natural sweetener
- 1 tbsp Unsweetened cocoa powder

Directions:

1. Remove the butter and cream cheese from the fridge for about 30 minutes before time to prepare to become room temperature. Chill a bowl and whisk the cream. Place back in the refrigerator for now.

2. Use a hand mixer to combine the sweetener, cream cheese, cocoa powder, and butter until well mixed. Remove the refrigerated cream and fold it into the chocolate mixture using a rubber scraper.

3. Portion it into two dessert bowls and chill for one hour.

Nutrition:

4g Protein

50g Total Fats

460 Calories

Chocolate Muffins

Preparation Time: 20 minutes

Cooking Time: 5 minutes

Servings: 6

Ingredients:

- ½ cup Coconut oil
- ½ cup Peanut butter
- Liquid stevia granulated sweetener (to your liking)

Directions:

1. Prepare the tin of choice with a spritz of oil. Combine the oil and peanut butter together on the stovetop or microwave. Melt and add the sweetener. Scoop into the tins or loaf pan and freeze.
2. You can serve with a drizzle of melted chocolate – but remember to count the carbs.

Nutrition:

7g Protein

14g Total Fats

193 Calories

Cannoli Dessert Dip

Preparation Time: 10 minutes

Cooking Time: 10 minutes

Servings: 8

Ingredients:

- ¾ cup (6 oz.) of softened Cream Cheese
- 1 cup of whole-milk Ricotta Cheese at room temp
- ½ tsp. of Vanilla extract
- ¾ cup of powdered Erythritol-based Sweetener, plus an additional amount for sprinkling
- 1/3 cup Sugarless Chocolate Chips
- ½ cup of heavy Whipping Cream

Directions:

1. Blend the vanilla extract, sweetener, cream cheese, and ricotta in a food processor or blender until smooth.
2. Whisk in the cream using an electric mixer in a medium bowl until it holds solid peaks. Carefully fold in the chocolate chips and the ricotta mixture and save some for later to sprinkle on top

Nutrition:

17.9g fats

5.6g Carbohydrates

5.7g protein

219 Calories

Slow Cooker Coffee Coconut Custard

Preparation Time: 5 minutes

Cooking Time: 2 hours

Servings: 4

Ingredients:

- 1 large egg
- 2 tbsp. of plus 1 cup of Full-Fat Coconut Milk
- ½ tsp. of Vanilla extract
- 2 large egg yolks
- 1 tsp. of Espresso powder
- ½ cup of powdered Erythritol-based Sweetener

Directions:

1. Whisk all the ingredients in a medium bowl until the espresso powder dissolves. Pour into 4-oz. coffee cups or ramekins and place in a slow cooker.
2. Fill up the slow cooker with water so that it goes halfway up the edges of the ramekins. Do not allow water to get into the custard.
3. Place over high heat for 1½-2 hours and stop when the middle is lightly jiggly but the custard is set.

4. Remove from the heat and allow to cool to room temp. Afterwards, refrigerate for 2 hours. Remove and serve.

Nutrition:

16.8g Fats

2.6g Carbohydrates

4.3g Protein

186 Calories

Coconut Lime Panna Cotta

Preparation Time: 10 minutes

Cooking Time: 5 minutes

Servings: 4

Ingredients:

- 1½ tsp. of grass-fed Gelatin
- 13.5-oz. (or 1) of can Full-Fat Coconut Milk
- 1 tsp. of grated Lime Zest
- 1/3 cup of powdered Erythritol-based Sweetener
- ¼ tsp. of Coconut extract
- 2 tbsp. of fresh Lime Juice

Directions:

1. Grease four 4-oz. ramekins. Whisk in the gelatin plus half of the coconut milk in a saucepan and place over medium heat. Allow to simmer and keep whisking until the gelatin dissolves.
2. Remove from heat and add the coconut extract, lime juice, lime zest, sweetener, and the rest of the coconut milk. Whisk to mix thoroughly and dissolve the sweetener.
3. Divide the mixture between the greased ramekins to refrigerate for 3 hours until it sets.

4. Place the ramekins in a dish of hot water for 20-30 seconds to unmold. Position the plate upside down on the top of the ramekins and turn everything over. Shake it thoroughly to free it

Nutrition:

18.5g Fats

3.2g Carbohydrates

2.6g protein

193 Calories

Chocolate Cobbler

Preparation Time: 10 minutes

Cooking Time: 40 minutes

Servings: 8

Ingredients:

Chocolate Layer Ingredients:

- 1/3 cup granulated Erythritol-based Sweetener
- 1¼ cups blanched Almond flour
- ¼ cup Cocoa powder
- 3 tbsp. of unflavored Whey Protein powder
- 2 tsp. of baking powder
- ½ tsp. of Espresso powder
- ¼ tsp. of salt
- ½ stick (¼ cup) of unsalted melted Butter
- ½ cup of heavy Whipping Cream

Topping Ingredients:

- 1 tbsp. of Cocoa powder
- ¾ cup of hot Water
- 2 tbsp. of granulated Erythritol-based Sweetener

Directions:

1. Heat the oven to 325° F. Preparing the chocolate layer: Whisk the baking powder, salt, espresso powder, protein powder, cocoa

powder, sweetener, and almond flour in a large bowl until it is well mixed. In an 8-inch baking dish, evenly spread the mixture.

2. Preparing the topping: Whisk the cocoa powder and the sweetener together in a small bowl. Evenly sprinkle on the top of the cobbler. Empty the hot water over the cobbler and make sure not to stir.
3. Place in an oven and bake for 35-40 minutes until the center is set.
4. Take out of the oven and allow to cool for 10-15 minutes. Serve warm.

Nutrition:

20g Fats

7.1g Carbohydrates

6.5g Protein

223 Calories

Easy Shortbread Crust

Preparation Time: 5 minutes

Cooking Time: 15 minutes

Servings: 10

Ingredients:

- ¼ cup of powdered Erythritol-based Sweetener
- 150g (1½ cups) of blanched Almond flour
- ¼ cup (½ stick) of unsalted melted Butter
- ½ tsp. of salt

Directions:

1. Whisk together the salt, sweetener, and almond flour in a medium dish.
2. Add the melted butter and stir until mixture starts to clump together.

Nutrition:

12.7g fats

3.6g Carbohydrates

3.7g Protein

137 Calories

Ketogenic Chocolate Kisses

Preparation Time: 10 minutes

Cooking Time: 15 minutes

Servings: 20

Ingredients:

- 2 ounces unsweetened baking chocolate
- 1 ½ tablespoons Swerve confectioners' powdered sweetener
- ¼ teaspoon vanilla extract
- A pinch stevia concentrated powder
- ½ ounce food grade cocoa butter

Directions:

1. Add chocolate, sweetener and cocoa butter into a heatproof bowl. Place the bowl in a double boiler. Stir occasionally until the mixture melts. You can also melt it in a small pan over low heat.
2. Add stevia and vanilla and mix well. Spoon into 20 chocolate molds. Cool completely.
3. Chill until firm. Remove from mold and serve. Leftovers can be stored in an airtight container in the refrigerator.

Nutrition:

24.8 Calories

08.g Carbohydrates

0.4g Protein

Ultra-Decadent

Chocolate Truffles

Preparation Time: 15 minutes

Cooking Time: 5 minutes

Servings: 20

Ingredients:

- 2 cups coconut cream
- 6-8 tablespoons cocoa powder + extra to dust
- ½ teaspoon kosher salt
- 4-8 tablespoons xylitol or Allulose or any other Ketogenic friendly sweetener
- ½ teaspoon espresso powder (optional)
- ½ teaspoon xanthan gum

Directions:

1. Place the saucepan over medium flame. Simultaneously, blend with an immersion blender until smooth. Dust with xanthan gum and continue blending until well incorporated and free from lumps.

2. If you find that the mixture is very thick and you are not able to stir easily, add water, a teaspoon at a time and mix well each time. The mixture should be thick enough for you to

shape into truffles so add water only if necessary.

3. Turn off the heat and transfer into a bowl. Cool for a while and cover with cling wrap. Place in the refrigerator until it sets. Make small balls of the mixture of 1-inch diameter.

4. Place some cocoa powder on a plate. Dredge your palms in cocoa powder and roll the balls so that the balls are lightly covered with cocoa. Be quick in doing this or else the balls will start coming back to room temperature. When that happens, they will start losing their shape and you will not be able to dredge. You can also remove a few at a time from the refrigerator and place them back in the refrigerator when done.

5. Transfer into an airtight container. These can last for a week.

Nutrition:

53.1 Calories

4.4g fats

1.1g Carbohydrates

0.8g Protein

CBD Chocolate

Coconut Fat Bombs

Preparation Time: 5 minutes

Cooking Time: 2 minutes

Servings: 10-12

Ingredients:

- ¼ cup CBD coconut oil
- ½ tablespoon Brothers Apothecary Wild Rosin Honey
- ¼ cup plain coconut butter (without CBD)

Directions:

1. Add coconut oil, CBD honey and coconut butter into a microwave safe bowl. Microwave on high in increments of 30 seconds. Stir every 30 seconds until the mixture melts and is smooth.
2. Pour into gummy molds. Let it cool for a few minutes. Chill until firm. Remove from mold and serve. Store in an airtight container in the refrigerator. These can keep for a week.

Nutrition:

101 Calories

10.25g Fats

2.25g Carbohydrates

0.33g protein

Ketogenic White Chocolate

Preparation Time: 10 minutes

Cooking Time: 15 minutes

Servings: 6

Ingredients:

- 16 ounces raw cacao butter
- 1 tablespoon dried cranberries (optional)
- 1-2 tablespoons chopped nuts of your choice (optional)
- Cayenne pepper
- 8-10 tablespoons Swerve or powdered erythritol
- 1 teaspoon vanilla extract
- ¾ teaspoon vanilla liquid stevia

Directions:

1. Place a saucepan over low heat. Add cacao butter into it. When it melts, turn off heat. You can also melt it in a double boiler. Add Swerve and whisk well.

2. Line 2 baking sheets with parchment paper. Divide the mixture between the baking sheets. Sprinkle cranberries, cayenne pepper and nuts if using and press lightly into the chocolate mixture. Chill until firm.

3. Break or chop into pieces. Transfer into an airtight container and refrigerate until use.

Nutrition:

1936 Calories

208g fats

4g Carbohydrates

Frozen Chocolate Roll

Preparation Time: 5 minutes

Cooking Time: 10 minutes

Servings: 8

Ingredients:

- 1 cup raw pecans
- 1-ounce unsweetened baking chocolate
- ½ tablespoon vanilla extract
- ½ cup grated or shredded coconut, unsweetened
- 1 ½ tablespoons Swerve or 2 teaspoons green stevia

Directions:

1. Add pecans, chocolate, vanilla, coconut and sweetener into the food processor bowl. Process until well incorporated.
2. Place a sheet of parchment paper on your countertop. Place the mixture on the parchment paper. Roll into a log with the help of the parchment paper.
3. Wrap the log with parchment paper and freeze until firm. Place on your cutting board. Unwrap and cut into ½ inch thick slices.

4. Serve immediately or transfer into a freezer safe container and freeze until use.

Nutrition:

144 Calories

14g Fats

4.35g Carbohydrates

2g Protein

Chocolaty Peanut Butter Cups

Preparation Time: 60 minutes

Cooking Time: 5 minutes

Servings: 6

Ingredients:

- 4 tbsp Nut butter
- 1 stick Unsalted butter
- 1 oz Unsweetened dark chocolate
- 1/3 cup Stevia/Monk fruit
- 2 tbsp Heavy cream

Directions:

1. Prepare a muffin tin with cupcake liner paper. Melt the butter and chocolate in the microwave (checking at 30-second intervals). Stir in the rest of the fixings.
2. Evenly distribute into the prepared tins and freeze for 30 minutes to an hour. Gently tap the pan to remove.

Nutrition:

1g Carbohydrates

2g Protein Counts

26g Total Fats

Coconut Bars

Preparation Time: 10 minutes

Cooking Time: 0 minute

Servings: 20

Ingredients:

- 3 cups Unsweetened shredded coconut
- 1 cup Coconut oil
- ¼ cup Liquid sweetener of choice

Directions:

1. Line a pan with a layer of parchment paper. Combine the ingredients to make a thick batter. Pour into the pan and freeze until firm. Cut into squares and store until you want a delicious snack.

Nutrition:

2g Protein

11g Total Fats

108 Calories

Coconut Cranberry Crack Bars

Preparation Time: 15 minutes

Cooking Time: 0 minute

Servings: 20

Ingredients:

- 2 ½ cups Unsweetened shredded coconut flakes
- ½ cup Unsweetened cranberries
- ¼ cup Monk fruit sweetened maple syrup/agave/pure maple syrup
- 1 cup Melted coconut oil

Directions:

1. Using a high-speed blender/food processor to combine the berries and coconut, pulsing until it's crumbly. Combine all of the fixings until thoroughly mixed. Pour the batter into the pan and refrigerate until firm. Slice into bars and add a bar of optional chocolate to your liking.
2. They're okay in the fridge for up to two months.

Nutrition:

2g Protein

9g Total Fats

98 Calories

Crunchy Berry Mousse

Preparation Time: 20 minutes

Cooking Time: 0 minute

Servings: 8

Ingredients:

- 2 cups Heavy whipping cream
- ¼ tsp Vanilla extract
- Lemon zest
- 2 oz. Chopped pecans
- 3 oz Fresh raspberries/blueberries/strawberries

Directions:

1. Use a hand mixer to whip the cream until it forms soft peaks. Then, add the vanilla and lemon zest.
2. Fold in the nuts and berries. Stir. Cover with a layer of plastic wrap. For a firmer mousse, store in the fridge for about four hours. You can enjoy it when freshly prepared if you like it less firm.

Nutrition:

3g Protein

27g Total Fats

260 Calories

Hot Chocolate Ice Cream

Preparation Time: 45 minutes

Cooking Time: 0 minute

Servings: 12

Ingredients:

- 2 cans Chilled coconut milk
- 1-4 scoops Chocolate protein powder
- 2 tbsp Cocoa powder
- 2 tbsp Granulated sweetener - ex. Monk fruit

Directions:

1. Put the pan in the freezer to chill. Take the can of milk out of the fridge and split the water from the cream. Add the cream into a food processor or high-speed blender, followed by the coconut water. Blend until just combined.
2. Add the protein powder, granulated sweetener, and cocoa powder. Blend until it's thick and creamy, but don't over-blend. Add the ice cream to the chilled pan. Lightly stir the ice cream every 20-30 minutes for the first hour to help prevent it from becoming too icy. When it's time to serve, thaw the loaf pan for approximately 15 minutes

Nutrition:

7g Protein

11g Total Fats

130 Calories

Low-Carb Cheesecake

Preparation Time: 10 minutes

Cooking Time: 20 minutes

Servings: 5

Ingredients:

- 8 oz room temp full-fat cream cheese
- 2 Large eggs
- 1 ½ tsp Granulated stevia/erythritol blend
- ¼ tsp Pure vanilla extract
- ¼ tsp Pure almond extract

Directions:

1. Warm the oven to 325° Fahrenheit. Prepare five muffin tin cups using cupcake liners. Beat the cream cheese until its creamy smooth, whisk in the eggs, and the rest of the fixings.

2. Dump the batter into the muffin tins. Set the timer (15-20 minutes.), and bake until the cheesecakes are puffy but still wobbly in the center.

3. Cool to room temperature before placing it in the refrigerator to chill for two hours before serving.

Nutrition:

4g Protein

17g Total Fats

181 Calories

Peanut Butter Fudge

Preparation Time: 9 minutes

Cooking Time: 31 minutes

Servings: 20

Ingredients:

- 3 tbsp Coconut oil
- 12 oz. Smooth peanut butter - Ketogenic-friendly
- 4 tbsp Coconut cream
- 4 tbsp Maple syrup
- Pinch of Salt

Directions:

1. Prepare a baking sheet with a layer of parchment paper. Melt the syrup and coconut oil using the medium heat setting on the stovetop. Stir in the salt, coconut cream, and peanut butter. Pour the mixture into the prepared dish and chill in the fridge for at least one hour. Slice into pieces and store or serve.

Nutrition:

4g Protein

11g Total Fats

135 Calories

Peanut Butter Mousse

Preparation Time: 20 minutes

Cooking Time: 0 minute

Servings: 3

Ingredients:

- ½ cup Heavy whipping cream
- 4 oz room temp cream cheese
- ¼ cup Powdered Swerve Sweetener
- ¼ cup Sugar-free natural peanut butter
- ½ tsp Vanilla extract

Directions:

1. In a medium bowl, whip the cream until it creates stiff peaks. Set aside for now. In another mixing container, beat the cream cheese, sweetener, peanut butter, and vanilla. Add a pinch of salt if the peanut butter is unsalted. Mix until creamy smooth.

2. If your mixture is overly thick, add about two tablespoons of heavy cream to lighten it and continue mixing. Gently fold in the whipped cream. Spoon or use a piping tool to add it into dessert glasses.

3. Drizzle using a portion of low-carb chocolate sauce or other toppings, as desired. (Be sure to count the additional carbs.)

Nutrition:

301 Calories

5.9g Protein

26.5g Total Fats

Raspberry Chia Pudding

Preparation Time: 10 minutes

Cooking Time: 0 minute

Servings: 2

Ingredients:

- 4 tbsp Chia seeds
- ½ cup Raspberries
- 1 cup Coconut milk

Directions:

1. Pour the milk and raspberries into a blender. Pulse until smooth. Pour into the jars.
2. Fold in the chia seeds and stir. Secure the lid and shake. Store in the fridge for at least three hours before serving.

Nutrition:

38.8 Protein Counts

28.3g Total Fats

408 Calories

Raspberry Soft-Serve Ice Cream

Preparation Time: 60 minutes

Cooking Time: 0 minute

Servings: 5

Ingredients:

- 1 cup Heavy cream or coconut cream

- 2 cups Frozen raspberries
- 1/3 cup Powdered erythritol or any sweetener

Directions:

1. Pour the cream into a blender. Blend until stiff peaks form (You can also use a hand mixer if your blender isn't powerful enough to whip the cream).
2. Toss the frozen raspberries and sweetener into the blender. Puree until incorporated. Adjust the sweetener to taste if needed, and if added, puree again.
3. For firmer ice cream, run the mixture through an ice cream maker, or place in the freezer to firm up. Stir every 30-60 minutes for the first couple hours to break up any ice crystals.

Nutrition:

1g Protein

16g Total Fats

183 Calories

Squash Pudding

Preparation time: 5 minutes

Cooking time: 0 minute

Servings: 1

Ingredients:

- 1/2 cup water
- 2 cups squash
- 7 dates, pitted
- 2 tbsp. coconut oil, virgin
- 2 tbsp. peanut butter
- 1 small ginger cube
- 1/2 vanilla bean pod, scraped
- 1 1/2 tbsp. cloves

Directions:

1. Pour water into a food processor than all other ingredients. Process until a creamy texture.
2. Serve and enjoy!

Nutrition:

Calories: 703

Protein: 11 g.

Sugar: 45 g.

Fiber: 15 g

Delicious Ricotta Cake

Preparation Time: 10 minutes

Cooking Time: 45 minutes

Servings: 8

Ingredients:

- 2 eggs
- ½ cup erythritol
- ¼ cup coconut flour
- 15 oz. ricotta
- Pinch of salt

Directions:

1. Start oven then preheat to 350 F/ 180C. Spray 9-inch baking pan with cooking spray and set aside. In a bowl whisk egg. Combine all ingredients.
2. Transfer batter in prepared baking pan. Bake in preheated oven for 45 minutes. Remove baking pan from oven and allow cooling completely. Slice and serve.

Nutrition:

91 Calories

2.9g Net Carbs

3 g Protein

Chocó Coconut Cake

Preparation Time: 10 minutes

Cooking Time: 25 minutes

Servings: 9

Ingredients:

- 6 eggs
- 1 tsp. vanilla
- 3 oz. butter, melted
- 11.5 oz. heavy whipping cream
- 2 tsp. baking powder
- 3 oz. unsweetened cocoa powder
- 5 oz. erythritol
- oz. coconut flour

Directions:

1. Start oven then preheat to 350 F/ 180C. In a bowl, mix together coconut flour, butter, 5.5 oz. heavy whipping cream, eggs, baking powder 1.5 oz. cocoa powder, and 3 oz. erythritol until well combined. Bake in preheated oven for 25 minutes.
2. Remove cake from oven and allow cooling completely. In a large bowl, beat remaining heavy whipping cream, cocoa powder and erythritol until smooth. Spread the cream on

the cake evenly. Chill for 30 minutes. Slice and serve.

Nutrition:

282 Calories

26.1 Total Fat

5.1g Fiber

Fudgy Chocolate Cake

Preparation Time: 10 minutes

Cooking Time: 30 minutes

Servings: 12

Ingredients:

- 6 eggs
- 1 ½ cup erythritol
- ½ cup almond flour
- oz. butter, melted
- oz. unsweetened chocolate, melted
- Pinch of salt

Directions:

1. Turn the oven on and preheat to 350 F/ 180C. Grease 8-inch spring-form cake pan with butter and set aside. Beat eggs in a large bowl.
2. Add sweetener and stir well. Add melted butter, chocolate, almond flour, and salt and stir until combined. Bake for 30 minutes.
3. Remove cake from oven and allow cooling completely. Slice and serve.

Nutrition:

360 Calories

37.6g Total Fat

4.6g Fiber

Cinnamon Almond Cake

Preparation Time: 10 minutes

Cooking Time: 20 minutes

Servings: 6

Ingredients:

- 4 eggs
- 1 teaspoon orange zest
- 2/3 cup dried cranberries
- 1 ½ cups almond flour
- 1 tsp. vanilla extract
- 2 tsp. mixed spice
- 2 tsp. cinnamon
- ¼ cup erythritol
- 1 cup butter, softened

Directions:

1. Turn the oven on and preheat to 350 F/ 180C. In a bowl, add sweetener and melted butter and beat until fluffy. Add cinnamon, vanilla, and mixed spice and stir well.

2. Add egg one by one and stir until well combined. Add almond flour, orange zest, and cranberries and mix until well combined. Pour batter in a greased cake pan and bake in preheated oven for 20 minutes. Slice and serve.

Nutrition:

484 Calories

47.6g Total Fat

3.9g Fiber

Lemon Cake

Preparation Time: 10 minutes

Cooking Time: 60 minutes

Servings: 10

Ingredients:

- 4 eggs
- 2 tbsp. lemon zest
- ½ cup fresh lemon juice
- ¼ cup erythritol
- 1 tbsp. vanilla
- ½ cup butter softened
- 2 tsp. baking powder
- ¼ cup coconut flour
- 2 cups almond flour

Directions:

1. Start oven and preheat to 300 F/ 150 C. Grease 9-inch loaf pan with butter and set aside. Combine all ingredients. Bake for 60 minutes. Slice and serve.

Nutrition:

244 Calories

22.3g Total Fat

2.7g Fiber

www.ingramcontent.com/pod-product-compliance
Lightning Source LLC
Chambersburg PA
CBHW061004050726

47592CB00003B/1334